CHRONIC KIDNEY DISEASE DIET COOKBOOK FOR BEGINNERS

A COMPREHENSIVE RECIPE, NUTRITION, AND MEAL PLANNING GUIDE TO EFFECTIVELY MANAGE AND SLOW THE PROGRESSION OF CHRONIC KIDNEY DISEASE THROUGH KIDNEY

Kirby Newlin

TABLE OF CONTENT

INTRODUCTION

Living with continual kidney ailment (CKD) presents specific demanding situations, in particular when it comes to food regimen and vitamins. What we devour has a profound impact on our health, and for those with CKD, making the right dietary selections can sluggish the development of the sickness, control symptoms, and improve normal nicely being. This cookbook goals to offer practical steering and delicious recipes tailored particularly for people with CKD, making it less complicated to navigate these dietary needs.

IMPORTANCE OF DIET IN MANAGING CKD

A well balanced weight loss program is vital for dealing with CKD. Proper nutrients allows manage blood strain, reduce the buildup of waste products within the blood, and maintain fluid stability. By focusing on the right foods and fending off the ones which can exacerbate kidney problems, individuals with CKD can notably enhance their firstrate of lifestyles.

GOALS OF THE COOKBOOK

This cookbook is designed with novices in mind, supplying truthful, clean to observe recipes and meal plans that align with CKD nutritional hints. Our goals are to:

Educate: Provide a clear expertise of the way distinctive nutrients have an effect on kidney health.

Simplify: Make meal making plans and preparation reachable and attainable.

Inspire: Show that a CKD pleasant food plan can be numerous, flavorful, and exciting.

Support: Offer practical recommendations and resources for coping with CKD through eating regimen.

UNDERSTANDING CHRONIC KIDNEY DISEASE

Chronic kidney sickness is a gradual loss of kidney characteristic over the years. The kidneys play a essential role in filtering waste and extra fluids from the blood, and when they're not functioning well, it can cause a buildup of harmful materials inside the body.

WHAT IS CKD?

CKD is classified into five degrees, with level 1 being the mildest and degree 5 being the maximum extreme, frequently requiring dialysis or a kidney transplant. The progression via those tiers can range substantially amongst individuals.

Stages of CKD

Stage 1: Mild kidney harm with ordinary or excessive kidney function.

Stage 2: Mild loss of kidney feature.

Stage 3: Moderate loss of kidney characteristic.

Stage four: Severe lack of kidney feature.

Stage 5: End level renal disorder (ESRD), requiring dialysis or transplant.

IMPORTANCE OF DIET IN MANAGING CKD

Managing continual kidney disorder (CKD) calls for a multifaceted approach, with food plan playing a pivotal role. The foods we eat at once affect kidney function and normal health, making nutritional selections a crucial component of CKD control. Understanding and imposing the proper nutritional strategies can help sluggish disorder progression, lessen signs and symptoms, and enhance first class of life.

CONTROLLING BLOOD PRESSURE

High blood strain is each a motive and a consequence of CKD. A food plan low in sodium can help manipulate blood strain stages, decreasing stress on the kidneys.

REDUCING WASTE PRODUCT BUILDUP

Healthy kidneys filter waste merchandise from the blood, however in CKD, this method is impaired. A CKD friendly eating regimen makes a speciality of lowering the intake of waste generating nutrients, which include phosphorus and potassium. By carefully dealing with those nutrients, patients can assist limit the buildup of dangerous materials in their blood, easing the workload on their kidneys.

MAINTAINING FLUID BALANCE

Proper hydration is vital for kidney health, but for CKD patients, it's critical to manipulate fluid intake to prevent headaches including swelling and excessive blood stress. A CKD eating regimen includes recommendations for fluid consumption, making sure that patients stay hydrated without overloading their kidneys.

SUPPORTING NUTRIENT NEEDS

CKD can alter the frame's potential to system and maintain positive vitamins, leading to deficiencies or imbalances. A carefully planned food regimen can provide the necessary nutrients and minerals even as warding off excesses which could damage the kidneys. This stability is crucial for preserving ordinary health and stopping additional health issues.

MANAGING SYMPTOMS AND COMPLICATIONS

Diet plays a sizable role in handling commonplace CKD symptoms together with fatigue, nausea, and muscle cramps. By following a CKD friendly weight loss plan, patients can alleviate those symptoms and prevent complications like bone ailment and cardiovascular troubles.

ENHANCING QUALITY OF LIFE

Adopting a CKD pleasant weight reduction plan not simplest facilitates control the ailment but additionally complements the patient's high quality of existence. Enjoying quite a few flavorful, nutritious ingredients can enhance temper, strength ranges, and usual nicely being. This cookbook targets to reveal that a CKD weight reduction plan doesn't need to be restrictive or bland—it may be fulfilling and scrumptious.

KEY DIETARY COMPONENTS FOR CKD MANAGEMENT

1. Protein: Essential for body feature but need to be fed on in moderation. Choose wonderful assets like lean meats, fish, and plant based proteins.

2. Sodium: Limit consumption to govern blood strain and fluid balance. Avoid processed ingredients and use herbs and spices for taste.

3. Potassium: High tiers may be risky for CKD patients. Monitor intake of culmination, greens, and dairy products.

Four. Phosphorus: Excess phosphorus can weaken bones. Limit foods like dairy, nuts, and processed meals containing phosphate additives.

5. Fluids: Monitor intake to prevent fluid overload. Balance fluid consumption with the body's wishes and the kidneys' ability.

COMMON SYMPTOMS AND COMPLICATIONS OF CKD

Chronic kidney ailment (CKD) often progresses slowly, and plenty of human beings won't revel in significant symptoms until the sickness is superior. Understanding the not unusual signs and symptoms and capacity complications of CKD can help in handling the situation effectively and searching for timely scientific intervention.

COMMON SYMPTOMS OF CKD

1. Fatigue

Description: Feeling tired or exhausted all of the time.

Cause: The buildup of waste products within the blood, anemia, and the frame's extended attempt to clear out blood.

2. Swelling (Edema)

Description: Swelling within the legs, ankles, feet, and occasionally the hands and face.

Cause: Fluid retention due to the kidneys' lack of ability to remove excess fluid.

3. Shortness of Breath

Description: Difficulty respiratory or feeling quick of breath.

Cause: Fluid buildup inside the lungs (pulmonary edema) or anemia.

4. Nausea and Vomiting

Description: Feeling ill to the belly and vomiting.

Cause: The accumulation of waste products and pollution within the blood.

5. Loss of Appetite

Description: Reduced choice to devour, main to weight loss.

Cause: The buildup of waste products and modifications in metabolism.

6. Changes in Urination

Description: Increased or decreased urination, changes in urine colour, or foamy urine.

Cause: The kidneys' impaired potential to filter and manner urine.

7. Muscle Cramps

Description: Painful cramps, mainly inside the legs.

Cause: Imbalances in electrolytes such as calcium, potassium, and magnesium.

8. Itchy Skin

Description: Persistent itching, regularly worse at night.

Cause: Accumulation of waste merchandise and excessive stages of phosphorus inside the blood.

9. High Blood Pressure (Hypertension)

Description: Elevated blood stress readings.

Cause: Fluid retention and hormonal imbalances affecting blood strain law.

10. Difficulty Concentrating

Description: Trouble focusing or experiencing intellectual fog.

Cause: Anemia and the accumulation of pollution affecting mind feature.

COMMON COMPLICATIONS OF CKD

1. Anemia

Description: A situation where there aren't enough purple blood cells to carry oxygen all through the frame.

Cause: Reduced manufacturing of erythropoietin, a hormone produced by means of the kidneys that stimulates purple blood cell manufacturing.

2. Bone Disease

Description: Weakening of bones, leading to fractures and bone pain.

Cause: Imbalances in calcium and phosphorus degrees, and reduced activation of diet D through the kidneys.

3. Cardiovascular Disease

Description: Increased hazard of coronary heart ailment, heart assaults, and strokes.

Cause: High blood pressure, excessive ranges of waste merchandise, and imbalances in electrolytes.

4. Fluid Overload

Description: Excess fluid within the body, main to swelling and heart failure.

Cause: The kidneys' incapacity to take away excess fluid from the frame.

5. Electrolyte Imbalances

Description: Abnormal tiers of electrolytes consisting of potassium, sodium, and calcium.

Cause: The kidneys' impaired capacity to balance electrolyte degrees.

6. High Potassium Levels (Hyperkalemia)

Description: Elevated ranges of potassium within the blood, that may affect coronary heart function.

Cause: Reduced kidney feature and the incapacity to excrete potassium well.

7. Metabolic Acidosis

Description: Increased acidity inside the blood.

Cause: The kidneys' reduced capacity to get rid of acid from the blood.

8. Uremia

Description: A intense buildup of waste merchandise inside the blood.

Cause: Advanced kidney failure.

CHAPTER 1: BASICS OF A CKD DIET

NUTRITIONAL NEEDS FOR CKD PATIENTS

PROTEIN

Protein is an vital nutrient for the frame's increase, restore, and typical function. However, for people with continual kidney disorder (CKD), managing protein consumption is essential. The kidneys play a substantial position in processing and filtering waste merchandise from protein metabolism.

THE ROLE OF PROTEIN INSIDE THE BODY

- Growth and Repair: Protein is vital for constructing and repairing tissues, along with muscle mass, pores and skin, and organs.

- Enzyme and Hormone Production: Many enzymes and hormones are proteins or depend upon proteins to characteristic properly.

- Immune Function: Proteins are important additives of the immune gadget, assisting to defend the frame from infections.

PROTEIN NEEDS FOR CKD PATIENTS

For CKD patients, protein needs range relying at the degree of the disorder. The goal is to balance enough protein consumption for physical functions whilst minimizing the stress on the kidneys.

1. Early Stages of CKD (Stages 13)

- Moderate Protein Intake: Patients can be cautioned to consume a mild quantity of protein. The consciousness is on exceptional protein assets to satisfy dietary desires without overloading the kidneys.

- Guidelines: Typically, 0.6 to zero.8 grams of protein according to kilogram of body weight in step with day.

2. Advanced Stages of CKD (Stages four5)

- Reduced Protein Intake: As kidney feature declines, protein intake is frequently further decreased to lower the weight on the kidneys.

- Guidelines: Usually, 0.6 grams of protein consistent with kilogram of frame weight in keeping with day, but particular desires ought to be individualized based totally on medical recommendation.

3. Dialysis Patients

- Increased Protein Needs: Dialysis gets rid of waste products however additionally filters out some protein, growing the need for better protein intake.

Guidelines: Generally, 1.2 to one.5 grams of protein per kilogram of frame weight in line with day to make amends for protein losses at some stage in dialysis.

HIGH QUALITY PROTEIN SOURCES

Choosing extraordinary protein sources is crucial for CKD sufferers. These resources offer crucial amino acids and are less complicated for the frame to make use of.

1. Animal Based Proteins

- Lean Meats: Chicken, turkey, and lean cuts of red meat or red meat.
- Fish: Salmon, tuna, and other low mercury fish, rich in omega3 fatty acids.
- Eggs: A versatile protein supply; egg whites are specially useful as they comprise much less phosphorus.

2. Plant Based Proteins

- Legumes: Beans, lentils, and chickpeas, even though they have to be fed on carefully due to their potassium and phosphorus content material.

- Tofu and Tempeh: Soyprimarily based proteins which are low in phosphorus.
- Nuts and Seeds: Almonds, chia seeds, and flax seeds, but element manage is important because of their excessive potassium content.

SODIUM

Sodium is a mineral important for preserving fluid stability, nerve feature, and muscle contractions. However, for individuals with continual kidney ailment (CKD), coping with sodium intake is essential to save you headaches such as excessive blood stress, fluid retention, and further kidney harm.

THE ROLE OF SODIUM WITHIN THE BODY

Fluid Balance: Sodium allows alter the amount of water in and round cells.

Nerve Function: Sodium is important for the transmission of nerve impulses.

Muscle Function: Sodium is involved in muscle contraction and rest.

WHY SODIUM MANAGEMENT IS IMPORTANT FOR CKD

For CKD sufferers, the kidneys' capacity to excrete excess sodium is impaired. This can cause several problems:

High Blood Pressure (Hypertension): Excess sodium can growth blood strain, which further damages the kidneys and hurries up the development of CKD.

Fluid Retention: High sodium consumption can purpose the body to hold fluid, main to swelling (edema) within the legs, ankles, and around the eyes.

Heart Strain: Both high blood stress and fluid retention positioned more strain at the heart, growing the threat of coronary heart ailment.

Recommended Sodium Intake for CKD

General Guidelines: It is generally endorsed that CKD sufferers restrict their sodium intake to less than 2,three hundred milligrams (mg) consistent with day. In extra superior stages of CKD, a stricter limit of one,500 mg in step with day can be advised.

Individualized Plans: Sodium wishes can vary based on the stage of CKD, presence of different health situations, and individual responses. Always consult a healthcare issuer or dietitian for customized recommendation.

TIPS FOR REDUCING SODIUM INTAKE

1. Choose Fresh and Unprocessed Foods

   Fresh fruits and veggies

   Fresh meats, fowl, and fish

   Whole grains like rice, quinoa, and oats

2. Read Nutrition Labels

- Look for products classified "low sodium," "sodium loose," or "no delivered salt."
- Check the sodium content material in step with serving and take note of serving sizes.

3. Cook at Home

- Preparing food at home permits better manage over the quantity of sodium in meals.
- Use sparkling ingredients and avoid adding salt for the duration of cooking.

4. Use Herbs and Spices

- Enhance the taste of meals with herbs, spices, garlic, lemon juice, and vinegar in preference to salt.
- Experiment with spice blends that don't comprise salt.

5. Limit Processed and Packaged Foods

● Avoid canned soups, processed meats (like bacon, ham, and sausage), frozen meals, and snack ingredients (like chips and pretzels) that are often excessive in sodium.

● Opt for low sodium variations of staples like canned beans and greens, rinsing them earlier than use.

6. Be Cautious with Condiments and Sauces

● Many condiments, sauces, and dressings are excessive in sodium.

● Choose low sodium versions or make your personal at domestic.

SODIUM SUBSTITUTES

● Avoid Salt Substitutes: Many salt substitutes include potassium chloride, which may be dangerous to CKD patients who want to display their potassium tiers.

- Natural Flavor Enhancers: Use options like garlic powder, onion powder, smoked paprika, and nutritional yeast to feature flavor with out more sodium.

POTASSIUM

Potassium is an critical mineral that performs a vital function in numerous bodily functions, including muscle contractions, nerve signaling, and retaining a ordinary heartbeat. For people with persistent kidney disorder (CKD), handling potassium intake is essential due to the kidneys' reduced capacity to regulate potassium tiers in the blood.

The Role of Potassium in the Body

Muscle Function: Potassium helps muscle tissue settlement and loosen up.

Nerve Function: It is critical for proper nerve signal transmission.

Heart Health: Potassium allows hold a ordinary heartbeat.

- Fluid and Electrolyte Balance: It enables stability fluids and electrolytes in the body.
- Why Potassium Management is Important for CKD
- As kidney feature declines, the kidneys turn out to be less green at removing excess potassium from the blood. High potassium stages (hyperkalemia) can cause critical fitness issues:
- Heart Problems: Elevated potassium ranges can cause irregular heartbeats (arrhythmias) and, in severe instances, can result in coronary heart assault.
- Muscle Weakness: High potassium can purpose muscle weak point and fatigue.
- Nerve Issues: It can affect nerve feature, main to tingling and numbness.

Recommended Potassium Intake for CKD

The advocated potassium consumption for CKD sufferers varies based totally on the level of the ailment, present day blood potassium levels, and general health:

General Guidelines: Typically, CKD sufferers are cautioned to devour among 2,000 to 3,000 milligrams (mg) of potassium in line with day. However, precise tips need to be individualized based totally on medical recommendation.

READING NUTRITION LABELS

Understanding and efficiently studying nutrients labels is crucial for dealing with a chronic kidney disease (CKD) diet. Labels provide crucial facts that allows you're making knowledgeable picks approximately the ingredients you devour, ensuring you adhere to nutritional restrictions and keep highest quality kidney health.

Key Components of Nutrition Labels

1. Serving Size

● Importance: The serving size on the pinnacle of the label suggests the amount of food the nutrients statistics are based on. It is essential to test this primary, as all of the dietary values at the label talk to this unique amount.

- Tip: Adjust the values as a result if you devour greater or much less than the said serving size.

2. Calories

- Importance: The quantity of energy in step with serving indicates the energy provided by way of the meals. Managing calorie intake is essential for keeping a healthful weight, in particular for CKD sufferers who may additionally need to keep away from excess weight gain.

3. Total Fat

- Importance: Includes the quantity of all varieties of fats in step with serving. Healthy fats are important, but CKD sufferers need to be cautious with saturated and trans fats to defend heart fitness.

- Tip: Look for meals low in saturated and trans fats.

4. Cholesterol

- Importance: Indicates the amount of cholesterol per serving. High ldl cholesterol intake can make a contribution to heart disorder, that's a not unusual hassle in CKD sufferers.

- Tip: Aim for ingredients with lower cholesterol levels.

5. Sodium

- Importance: Shows the quantity of sodium per serving. Managing sodium intake is crucial for controlling blood pressure and fluid stability in CKD.

- Tip: Choose foods with low sodium content, preferably less than a hundred and forty mg in line with serving for low sodium meals.

6. Total Carbohydrate

- Importance: Includes all types of carbohydrates, including sugars, fibers, and starches. Carbohydrates offer electricity, however coping with them is vital, specially when you have diabetes along with CKD.

- Tip: Pay attention to fiber content as nicely, which aids in digestion and typical health.

7. Dietary Fiber

- Importance: Part of total carbohydrates, fiber is crucial for digestive health and can help manipulate blood sugar stages.

- Tip: Choose foods high in fiber however low in potassium and phosphorus.

8. Sugars

- Importance: Indicates the quantity of natural and delivered sugars in line with serving. Excess sugar consumption can make a contribution to weight gain and get worse diabetes.

Tip: Opt for ingredients with low introduced sugar content material.

9. Protein

- Importance: Indicates the amount of protein in keeping with serving. CKD patients need to manipulate protein consumption primarily based on their degree of kidney disease.

- Tip: Balance protein consumption in line with nutritional recommendations.

CHAPTER 2: SETTING UP YOUR CKD FRIENDLY KITCHEN

ESSENTIAL TOOLS AND EQUIPMENT

CKD FRIENDLY INGREDIENTS

Choosing the proper ingredients is critical for dealing with chronic kidney ailment (CKD) via weight loss plan. CKD friendly substances assist manage potassium, phosphorus, sodium, and protein intake, making sure that meals are both nutritious and secure for kidney fitness.

FRUITS AND VEGETABLES

Low Potassium Fruits:

- Apples: Great for snacking or including to salads.
- Berries: Strawberries, blueberries, raspberries, and blackberries are outstanding low potassium alternatives.

- Grapes: Can be eaten fresh or added to salads.

- Pears: A flexible fruit that can be eaten fresh or cooked.

- Pineapple: Fresh or canned in juice, no longer syrup.

Low Potassium Vegetables:

- Cabbage: Can be used in salads, stir fries, or soups.

- Cauliflower: Versatile for roasting, mashing, or adding to dishes.

- Cucumbers: Great for salads and snacks.

- Green Beans: Can be steamed, sauteed, or added to casseroles.

- Lettuce: Ideal for salads and sandwiches.

- Bell Peppers: Can be eaten uncooked, roasted, or stuffed.

Grains and Starches

White Rice: A staple grain that is low in potassium and phosphorus.

- Pasta: Choose ordinary pasta over whole grain to lessen phosphorus consumption.

- White Bread: Lower in potassium and phosphorus than entire grain bread.

- Tortillas: Opt for white flour tortillas over entire grain.

- Rice Cakes: A low potassium, low phosphorus snack option.

FOODS TO AVOID

For individuals with persistent kidney sickness (CKD), certain ingredients can exacerbate symptoms and headaches by way of contributing to the accumulation of waste products and imbalances in electrolytes. Avoiding or proscribing those meals is critical for managing CKD successfully.

High Potassium Foods

1. Bananas

Rich in potassium, which may be dangerous if fed on in extra.

2. Oranges and Orange Juice

- High in potassium and must be avoided or constrained.

- Three. Tomatoes and Tomato Based Products

- Include clean tomatoes, tomato sauce, and tomato juice.

4. Potatoes

Both white and sweet potatoes are excessive in potassium; if ate up, they have to be leached to lessen potassium content material.

5. Avocados

Very excessive in potassium.

6. Spinach and Swiss Chard

High in potassium, particularly whilst cooked.

High Phosphorus Foods

1. Dairy Products

Includes milk, cheese, yogurt, and ice cream.

2. Nuts and Seeds

Includes almonds, peanuts, and sunflower seeds.

3. Beans and Lentils

High in phosphorus and should be confined.

4. Whole Grains

Brown rice, whole wheat bread, and oatmeal are excessive in phosphorus.

5. Processed Meats

Such as bacon, sausage, and deli meats, often include phosphorus additives.

High Sodium Foods

1. Processed and Packaged Foods

Includes chips, pretzels, canned soups, and frozen dinners.

2. Cured Meats

Such as ham, bacon, sausage, and warm puppies.

3. Pickles and Olives

- High in sodium because of the brining method.

- Four. Salty Snacks

- Includes salted nuts, popcorn, and crackers.

CHAPTER 3: MEAL PLANNING AND PREP

CREATING A BALANCED CKD MEAL PLAN

BATCH COOKING AND MEAL PREP TIPS

Batch cooking and meal prepping can be notably helpful for individuals with continual kidney disease (CKD), taking into account higher manage over elements and portion sizes even as saving time and reducing pressure at some point of the week.

Planning Your Meals

1. Create a Weekly Menu

- Plan food that meet your nutritional wishes for the whole week.
- Include a whole lot of low potassium, low phosphorus, and occasional sodium options to hold food thrilling.

2. Make a Grocery List

- List all of the ingredients you'll want to your deliberate meals.

- Stick to the listing to avoid impulse purchases that may not be CKD friendly.

3. Choose Simple Recipes

- Opt for recipes that require minimal substances and steps.

- Look for dishes that can be without problems modified to suit your nutritional restrictions.

BATCH COOKING TIPS

1. Cook in Large Quantities

Prepare big batches of kidney pleasant staples like rice, pasta, and cooked veggies.

Use larger pots and pans to cook dinner multiple servings without delay.

2. Utilize Slow Cookers and Instant Pots

These home equipment can save time and effort, allowing you to prepare dinner food in bulk with out steady supervision.

3. Cook Protein Ahead of Time

Prepare and element out protein sources like hen, turkey, or fish.

Store them within the refrigerator or freezer for clean get admission to in the course of the week.

4. Double Up Recipes

When cooking, double the recipe to make certain you have got enough for a couple of meals.

Store leftovers in portion sized boxes.

WEEKLY MEAL PLAN

Here's a CKD pleasant weekly meal plan that focuses on balanced, low potassium, low phosphorus, and low sodium meals. This plan includes breakfast, lunch, dinner, and snacks to help control CKD efficaciously.

Monday

Breakfast:

Oatmeal with fresh berries (low potassium fruit like strawberries or blueberries)

Unsweetened almond milk

Lunch:

Chicken salad with lettuce, cucumbers, and bell peppers

Olive oil and vinegar dressing

Dinner:

Grilled salmon with white rice

Steamed green beans

Snack:

Rice cakes with a small amount of peanut butter (limit portion size)

Tuesday

Breakfast:

Scrambled eggs with chopped bell peppers and onions

Whole wheat toast (low sodium)

Lunch:

Turkey and cheese sandwich on white bread

Side of apple slices

Dinner:

Baked chicken breast with mashed cauliflower

Steamed carrots

Snack:

Fresh pineapple chunks

Wednesday

Breakfast:

Greek yogurt (low phosphorus) with clean strawberries

A small handful of almonds (restricted portion)

Lunch:

Quinoa salad with cucumbers, tomatoes (small quantity), and olive oil dressing

Hard boiled egg

Dinner:

Lean red meat chop with sauteed zucchini

Couscous

Snack:

Unsalted popcorn

Thursday

Breakfast:

Smoothie with unsweetened almond milk, berries, and a small quantity of spinach

Whole wheat toast (low sodium)

Lunch:

Tuna salad with blended veggies and cucumbers

Olive oil and lemon juice dressing

Dinner:

Baked cod with roasted cauliflower

Brown rice

Snack:

Fresh pear slices

Friday

Breakfast:

Whole grain cereal (low sodium) with unsweetened almond milk

Fresh blueberries

Lunch:

Chicken wrap with lettuce, cucumbers, and bell peppers in a white flour tortilla

Side of sparkling grapes

Dinner:

Turkey meatloaf with mashed potatoes (leached to lessen potassium)

Steamed broccoli

Snack:

Carrot sticks with hummus

Saturday

Breakfast:

Pancakes made with white flour and crowned with clean berries

Unsweetened almond milk

Lunch:

Egg salad sandwich on white bread

Side of fresh pineapple chunks

Dinner:

Beef stir fry with bell peppers, snap peas, and carrots

White rice

Snack:

Rice desserts with a small quantity of peanut butter

Sunday

Breakfast:

Scrambled eggs with diced zucchini and onions

CHAPTER 4: BREAKFAST RECIPES

KIDNEY FRIENDLY SMOOTHIES

Low Sodium Breakfast Options
Maintaining a low sodium diet is vital for coping with continual kidney disease (CKD).

1. Oatmeal with Fresh Berries
Ingredients:
   1/2 cup old fashioned oats
   1 cup unsweetened almond milk
   Fresh berries (e.G., strawberries, blueberries)
   A sprinkle of cinnamon
Instructions:
   1. Cook oats in almond milk in step with package deal commands.
   2. Top with clean berries and a sprinkle of cinnamon.

2. Scrambled Eggs with Vegetables

Ingredients:

 2 massive eggs

 1/four cup chopped bell peppers

 1/four cup chopped onions

 1/4 cup chopped zucchini

 1 tsp olive oil

 Fresh floor black pepper to flavor

Instructions:

 1. Heat olive oil in a nonstick skillet over medium warmness.

 2. Add chopped veggies and saute till soft.

 Three. Whisk eggs in a bowl and pour over greens.

4. Cook, stirring frequently, until eggs are fully cooked.

 5. Season with black pepper to taste.

3. Greek Yogurt with Fruit and Nuts

 Ingredients:

1 cup undeniable Greek yogurt (low phosphorus)

Fresh fruit (e.G., berries, apple slices, pear slices)

1 tbsp chopped unsalted nuts (e.G., almonds, walnuts)

Instructions:

1. Top Greek yogurt with clean fruit and nuts.

2. Mix and revel in.

Protein Packed Breakfast Ideas

Protein Packed Breakfast Ideas

For people with persistent kidney disorder (CKD), balancing protein consumption is important.

1. Greek Yogurt Parfait

Ingredients:

1 cup simple Greek yogurt (low phosphorus)

half cup sparkling berries (e.G., strawberries, blueberries)

1 tbsp chia seeds or flax seeds

Instructions:

1. Layer Greek yogurt in a bowl or glass.

2. Top with fresh berries.

Three. Sprinkle chia seeds or flax seeds on pinnacle.

2. Scrambled Eggs with Spinach and Mushrooms

Ingredients:

2 massive eggs

half cup sparkling spinach leaves

1/four cup sliced mushrooms

1 tsp olive oil

Fresh floor black pepper to taste

Instructions:

1. Heat olive oil in a nonstick skillet over medium heat.

2. Add sliced mushrooms and cook dinner until they start to soften.

3. Add spinach leaves and cook till wilted.

4. Whisk eggs in a bowl and pour into the skillet.

5. Cook, stirring regularly, until eggs are completely cooked.

6. Season with black pepper to flavor.

3. Cottage Cheese and Fruit Bowl

Ingredients:

1 cup low sodium cottage cheese

Fresh fruit (e.G., pineapple chunks, peach slices, berries)

1 tbsp chia seeds or flax seeds

Instructions:

1. Scoop cottage cheese right into a bowl.

2. Top with fresh fruit.

Three. Sprinkle chia seeds or flax seeds on top.

4. Quinoa Breakfast Bowl

Ingredients:

half of cup cooked quinoa

1/4 cup low fats milk or unsweetened almond milk

1/4 cup clean berries

1 tbsp chopped nuts (e.G., almonds, walnuts)

A sprinkle of cinnamon

Instructions:

1. Warm cooked quinoa in a small saucepan with milk.

2. Transfer to a bowl and top with sparkling berries and chopped nuts.

3. Sprinkle with cinnamon.

5. Protein Smoothie

Ingredients:

1 cup unsweetened almond milk or low fats milk

half of cup plain Greek yogurt

half of cup frozen berries

1 tbsp chia seeds or flax seeds

1/2 banana (optionally available, if potassium consumption allows)

CHAPTER 5: LUNCH RECIPES

HEARTY SALADS

CKD FRIENDLY SANDWICHES AND WRAPS

Creating CKD friendly sandwiches and wraps entails deciding on substances which can be low in sodium, potassium, and phosphorus at the same time as still providing true flavor and nutrition.

1. Turkey and Cucumber Sandwich

Ingredients:

2 slices white bread (low sodium)

2 oz.Sliced turkey breast (low sodium, no brought preservatives)

1/four cup thinly sliced cucumber

1 leaf of lettuce

1 tbsp low fat mayonnaise or mustard (nonobligatory)

Instructions:

1. Spread mayonnaise or mustard on the bread if favored.

2. Layer turkey, cucumber slices, and lettuce on one slice of bread.

3. Top with the second one slice of bread and cut in half.

2. Chicken and Spinach Wrap

Ingredients:

1 massive white flour tortilla

3 oz.Cooked bird breast (shredded or sliced)

1/four cup sparkling spinach leaves

1/four cup diced pink bell pepper

1 tbsp low fat Greek yogurt (as a variety or dip)

Instructions:

1. Spread Greek yogurt at the tortilla.

2. Layer chook, spinach, and bell pepper on the tortilla.

3. Roll up the tortilla tightly and reduce in half of.

3. Egg Salad Sandwich

Ingredients:

2 slices white bread (low sodium)

2 difficult boiled eggs, chopped

1 tbsp low fat mayonnaise

1 tsp Dijon mustard

Fresh floor black pepper to taste

Instructions:

1. In a bowl, blend chopped eggs, mayonnaise, Dijon mustard, and pepper.

2. Spread the egg salad on one slice of bread.

3. Top with the second one slice of bread and cut in 1/2.

4. Tuna and Avocado Wrap

Ingredients:

1 massive white flour tortilla

1 can tuna packed in water, tired

1/four avocado, mashed

1/four cup shredded lettuce

1 tbsp low fat Greek yogurt or a small quantity of low sodium mayonnaise

Instructions:

1. Mix the tuna with Greek yogurt or mayonnaise.

2. Spread mashed avocado on the tortilla.

3. Layer the tuna combination and shredded lettuce on top.

4. Roll up the tortilla tightly and reduce in half of.

5. Hummus and Veggie Wrap

Ingredients:

1 big white flour tortilla

1/four cup hummus (low sodium, made from scratch or save bought without a introduced salt)

1/four cup thinly sliced bell peppers

1/4 cup thinly sliced cucumbers

1/4 cup shredded carrots

Instructions:

1. Spread hummus flippantly over the tortilla.

2. Layer bell peppers, cucumbers, and shredded carrots on top.

Three. Roll up the tortilla tightly and cut in half of.

6. Chicken Caesar Wrap

Ingredients:

1 big white flour tortilla

3 oz.Cooked hen breast, sliced

1/4 cup romaine lettuce

1 tbsp low sodium Caesar dressing

1 tbsp grated Parmesan cheese (non compulsory, in moderation)

SOUPS AND STEWS

CKD Friendly Soups and Stews

Soups and stews may be nourishing and comforting, in particular when tailor made to fulfill the nutritional needs of individuals with persistent kidney disorder (CKD).

1. Chicken and Vegetable Soup

Ingredients:

1 lb boneless, skinless chook breast, diced

4 cups low sodium fowl broth

1 cup diced carrots

1 cup diced celery

1 cup chopped cabbage

1 bay leaf

1 tsp dried thyme

Fresh ground black pepper to flavor

Instructions:

1. In a massive pot, deliver the fowl broth to a boil.

2. Add diced chook and cook dinner till not crimson.

3. Add carrots, celery, cabbage, bay leaf, and thyme.

4. Reduce heat and simmer until veggies are soft.

5. Season with black pepper to flavor. Remove bay leaf before serving.

2. Lentil and Vegetable Soup

Ingredients:

1 cup dried lentils, rinsed and drained

four cups low sodium vegetable broth

1 cup diced carrots

1 cup diced zucchini

1 cup chopped spinach

1 tsp cumin

Fresh ground black pepper to flavor

Instructions:

1. In a huge pot, deliver vegetable broth to a boil.

2. Add lentils and prepare dinner for 15 mins.

3. Add carrots, zucchini, and cumin. Simmer until lentils and greens are smooth.

Four. Stir in spinach and cook dinner till wilted.

5. Season with black pepper to flavor.

3. Turkey and Sweet Potato Stew

Ingredients:

1 lb ground turkey

4 cups low sodium fowl or vegetable broth

2 cups diced candy potatoes (leached to reduce potassium)

1 cup chopped green beans

1 cup diced tomatoes (small quantity for taste)

1 tsp dried rosemary

Fresh ground black pepper to flavor

Instructions:

1. In a massive pot, cook floor turkey over medium heat till browned. Drain excess fat.

2. Add broth, candy potatoes, inexperienced beans, tomatoes, rosemary, and black pepper.

3. Bring to a boil, then reduce heat and simmer till candy potatoes and green beans are gentle.

4. Beef and Barley Soup

Ingredients:

1 lb lean pork stew meat, diced

4 cups low sodium beef broth

half of cup pearl barley

1 cup diced carrots

1 cup chopped celery

1 bay leaf

1 tsp dried thyme

Fresh floor black pepper to flavor

Instructions:

1. In a massive pot, brown the red meat over medium warmness.

2. Add beef broth, barley, carrots, celery, bay leaf, and thyme.

3. Bring to a boil, then lessen heat and simmer until red meat and barley are smooth.

4. Season with black pepper to taste.

Remove bay leaf earlier than serving.

CHAPTER 6: DINNER RECIPES

EASY WEEKNIGHT DINNERS

CKD FRIENDLY ONE POT MEALS

One pot food are convenient and may be tailor made to in shape a CKD pleasant weight loss plan. They help reduce cleanup whilst permitting you to % in flavor and nutrients.

1. Chicken and Rice Skillet

Ingredients:

1 lb boneless, skinless fowl breasts, diced

1 cup white rice

2 cups low sodium bird broth

1 cup diced carrots

1 cup frozen peas

1 tbsp olive oil

1 tsp dried thyme

Fresh floor black pepper to taste

Instructions:

1. Heat olive oil in a massive skillet over medium heat. Add diced chook and cook till no longer crimson.

2. Add rice, bird broth, carrots, and thyme.

Three. Bring to a boil, then lessen warmth, cowl, and simmer for about 20 minutes, or till rice is cooked.

4. Stir in frozen peas and cook for any other 5 mins.

5. Season with black pepper to flavor.

2. Turkey and Vegetable Casserole

Ingredients:

1 lb floor turkey

1 cup diced zucchini

1 cup chopped bell peppers

1 cup cooked quinoa

2 cups low sodium vegetable broth

1 tsp dried basil

half of tsp garlic powder

Fresh ground black pepper to flavor

Instructions:

1. In a massive pot or Dutch oven, cook dinner ground turkey over medium warmness until browned. Drain excess fat.

2. Add zucchini, bell peppers, and quinoa. Stir to combine.

3. Pour in vegetable broth, basil, and garlic powder.

4. Bring to a boil, then lessen warmth, cover, and simmer for approximately 15 mins, or until veggies are gentle.

5. Season with black pepper to taste.

three. Beef and Barley Stew

Ingredients:

1 lb lean beef stew meat, diced

half cup pearl barley

1 cup diced carrots

1 cup chopped celery

four cups low sodium beef broth

1 tsp dried rosemary

1 tsp dried thyme

FRESH FLOOR BLACK PEPPER TO FLAVOR

Fresh Ground Black Pepper to Taste

Using clean floor black pepper can enhance the taste of your meals with out including sodium.

1. Start with a Small Amount

Recommendation: Begin with a small pinch of freshly ground black pepper. You can continually upload extra to taste, however it's simpler to feature greater than to eliminate it as soon as it's been brought.

2. Use a Pepper Mill

Advantage: A pepper mill permits you to grind clean peppercorns, which provides a greater severe and aromatic taste in comparison to preground pepper.

3. Pair with Other Herbs and Spices

Idea: To upload flavor without counting on salt, integrate black pepper with other CKD pleasant herbs and spices like basil, thyme, rosemary, or cumin. This can create a properly rounded flavor profile.

4. Adjust Based on Your Sensitivity Consideration: If you're touchy to spice or have unique nutritional regulations, begin with much less pepper and modify consistent with your taste possibilities and tolerances.

5. Use in Cooking and as a Finishing Touch Application:

- Cooking: Add a small amount of black pepper at the same time as cooking soups, stews, and casseroles.

- Finishing Touch: Sprinkle a bit of clean floor black pepper on completed dishes like salads, sandwiches, or grilled meats for a further taste boost.

Vegetarian and Vegan Options

CKD Friendly Vegetarian and Vegan Options

Vegetarian and vegan food can be nutritious and scrumptious even as accommodating CKD dietary restrictions.

1. Chickpea and Spinach Stew

Ingredients:

1 can chickpeas, drained and rinsed

1 cup chopped clean spinach

1 cup diced tomatoes (low potassium quantity)

1 cup low sodium vegetable broth

1 tsp dried oregano

1 tsp garlic powder

Fresh ground black pepper to flavor

Instructions:

1. In a big pot, heat vegetable broth over medium warmth.

2. Add diced tomatoes, chickpeas, oregano, and garlic powder.

3. Simmer for 10 mins.

4. Stir in clean spinach and cook until wilted.

5. Season with black pepper to flavor.

2. Quinoa and Vegetable Stir Fry

Ingredients:

1 cup cooked quinoa

1 cup diced bell peppers

1 cup chopped zucchini

1 cup snap peas

1 tbsp olive oil

1 tsp soy sauce (low sodium)

Fresh ground black pepper to flavor

Instructions:

1. Heat olive oil in a huge skillet or wok over medium excessive warmth.

2. Add bell peppers, zucchini, and snap peas. Stir fry till tender crisp.

3. Add cooked quinoa and soy sauce.

4. Stir to combine and heat through.

5. Season with black pepper to flavor.

3. Stuffed Bell Peppers

Ingredients:

four bell peppers, tops reduce off and seeds eliminated

1 cup cooked brown rice

half of cup diced tomatoes (low potassium quantity)

half of cup black beans, rinsed and tired

half cup corn kernels (clean or frozen)

1 tsp dried cumin

Fresh floor black pepper to flavor

Instructions:

1. Preheat oven to 375°F (one hundred ninety°C).

2. In a bowl, combine cooked rice, tomatoes, black beans, corn, and cumin.

3. Stuff the bell peppers with the combination.

4. Place in a baking dish and bake for 2530 minutes, or until peppers are soft.

5. Season with black pepper to taste.

4. Lentil and Carrot Soup

Ingredients:

1 cup dried lentils, rinsed and tired

4 cups low sodium vegetable broth

1 cup diced carrots

1 cup chopped celery

1 tsp dried thyme

Fresh floor black pepper to flavor

Instructions:

1. In a massive pot, bring vegetable broth to a boil.

2. Add lentils, carrots, celery, and thyme.

3. Reduce heat and simmer for 30 minutes, or till lentils and veggies are soft.

Four. Season with black pepper to taste.

5. Vegan Stuffed Sweet Potatoes

Ingredients:

4 medium sweet potatoes

1 can black beans, tired and rinsed

1 cup corn kernels (sparkling or frozen)

half cup diced pink bell peppers

1 tsp cumin

1 tbsp olive oil

Fresh floor black pepper to flavor

Instructions:

1. Preheat oven to 400°F (two hundred°C).

2. Pierce sweet potatoes with a fork and bake for forty five60 mins, or till tender.

Three. In a bowl, blend black beans, corn, bell peppers, cumin, and olive oil.

Four. Cut sweet potatoes open and fluff with a fork.

Five. Top with the bean mixture.

6. Season with black pepper to taste.

6. Cauliflower Rice and Vegetable Bowl

Ingredients:

1 head cauliflower, grated into rice sized portions

1 cup diced bell peppers

1 cup chopped broccoli

1 tbsp olive oil

CHAPTER 7: SNACKS AND APPETIZERS

HEALTHY SNACK IDEAS

KIDNEY FRIENDLY DIPS AND SPREADS

Creating tasty and kidney friendly dips and spreads involves the usage of low sodium, low potassium, and coffee phosphorus components.

1. Hummus

Ingredients:

    1 can chickpeas, drained and rinsed

    2 tbsp tahini (optional, use sparingly)

    2 tbsp olive oil

    1 clove garlic, minced

    Juice of 1 lemon

    1/2 tsp ground cumin

    Fresh floor black pepper to taste

Instructions:

1. In a food processor, integrate chickpeas, tahini (if the use of), olive oil, garlic, lemon juice, and cumin.

2. Blend till smooth. If the aggregate is simply too thick, add a bit water or extra olive oil to attain the desired consistency.

3. Season with black pepper to flavor.

2. Avocado and Lime Dip

Ingredients:

1 ripe avocado, mashed

Juice of one lime

1 small tomato, diced (optional, if potassium lets in)

1 tbsp chopped fresh cilantro

Fresh ground black pepper to taste

Instructions:

1. In a bowl, integrate mashed avocado, lime juice, diced tomato (if using), and cilantro.

2. Stir till well combined.

3. Season with black pepper to flavor.

3. Greek Yogurt and Cucumber Dip

Ingredients:

1 cup undeniable Greek yogurt (low phosphorus)

half cucumber, finely diced

1 tbsp chopped sparkling dill

1 clove garlic, minced

Fresh floor black pepper to taste

Instructions:

1. In a bowl, blend Greek yogurt, cucumber, dill, and garlic.

2. Stir till nicely blended.

3. Season with black pepper to taste.

4. Roasted Red Pepper Spread

Ingredients:

1 jar (about 12 ounces) roasted red peppers, tired

1 tbsp olive oil

1 clove garlic, minced

1 tsp dried basil

Fresh floor black pepper to taste

Instructions:

1. In a meals processor, integrate roasted pink peppers, olive oil, garlic, and basil.

2. Blend till clean.

3. Season with black pepper to flavor.

5. White Bean and Herb Spread

Ingredients:

1 can cannelloni beans, tired and rinsed

2 tbsp olive oil

1 tbsp chopped sparkling parsley

1 tbsp chopped fresh basil

Juice of half of lemon

Fresh ground black pepper to flavor

Instructions:

1. In a meals processor, integrate cannelloni beans, olive oil, parsley, basil, and lemon juice.

2. Blend till clean.

3. Season with black pepper to taste.

6. Apple and Celery Spread

Ingredients:

1 apple, peeled and finely diced

2 stalks celery, finely diced

2 tbsp low fats simple yogurt

1 tbsp chopped sparkling parsley

Fresh ground black pepper to taste

Instructions:

1. In a bowl, blend apple, celery, yogurt, and parsley.

2. Stir till properly combined.

3. Season with black pepper to taste.

LOW SODIUM APPETIZERS

Creating appetizers that are low in sodium at the same time as nevertheless being scrumptious and pleasurable is vital for a CKD friendly food regimen.

1. Cucumber and Hummus Bites

Ingredients:

1 cucumber, sliced into rounds

1/2 cup self made or low sodium keep bought hummus

Fresh dill or parsley for garnish

Instructions:

1. Spread a small quantity of hummus on every cucumber slice.

2. Garnish with clean dill or parsley.

3. Serve straight away.

2. Stuffed Mini Bell Peppers

Ingredients:

8 mini bell peppers, tops cut off and seeds removed

half cup low fat cream cheese or Greek yogurt

1 tbsp chopped clean chives

1 tsp dried oregano

Fresh ground black pepper to flavor

Instructions:

1. In a bowl, blend cream cheese (or Greek yogurt), chives, oregano, and black pepper.

2. Stuff every mini bell pepper with the mixture.

3. Chill earlier than serving.

three. Fresh Veggie Sticks with Greek Yogurt Dip

Ingredients:

1 cup undeniable Greek yogurt (low phosphorus)

1 tbsp chopped sparkling dill

1 tsp lemon juice

Fresh ground black pepper to taste

Assorted clean veggie sticks (carrots, celery, bell peppers)

Instructions:

1. In a bowl, mix Greek yogurt, dill, lemon juice, and black pepper.

2. Serve with sparkling veggie sticks.

4. Baked Sweet Potato Chips

Ingredients:

2 medium sweet potatoes, thinly sliced

1 tbsp olive oil

half of tsp paprika

Fresh ground black pepper to flavor

Instructions:

1. Preheat oven to 400°F (2 hundred°C).

2. Toss candy potato slices with olive oil, paprika, and black pepper.

3. Arrange in a single layer on a baking sheet.

4. Bake for 1520 minutes, or until crispy.

5. Tomato Basil Bruschetta

Ingredients:

1 cup diced tomatoes (low potassium quantity)

2 tbsp chopped fresh basil

1 tbsp balsamic vinegar

1 tbsp olive oil

Fresh floor black pepper to flavor

Wholegrain or low sodium baguette slices

Instructions:

1. In a bowl, integrate diced tomatoes, basil, balsamic vinegar, olive oil, and black pepper.

2. Spoon mixture onto baguette slices.

3. Serve right away.

6. Zucchini Roll Ups

Ingredients:

2 medium zucchinis, sliced lengthwise into thin strips

half cup low fats ricotta cheese or Greek yogurt

1 tbsp chopped clean basil

Fresh floor black pepper to flavor

www.ingramcontent.com/pod-product-compliance
Lightning Source LLC
Chambersburg PA
CBHW071952210526
45479CB00003B/905